FUTURISTIC CONCEPTS IN MEDICINE

BY DAVID LEFKON AND ARTIFICIAL INTELLIGENCE

TABLE OF CONTENTS

Introduction to Futuristic Concepts in Medicine 7
    The Medical Frontier 7
    The Potential Impact 8
    A New Age of Medicine 8
    Challenges and Opportunities 8
Artificial Intelligence in Medicine 10
    AI-Powered Diagnostics 10
    AI-Driven Treatment Planning 11
    Medical Research and Drug Discovery 11
    AI in Patient Care 12
    Challenges and Ethical Considerations 12
Gene Editing 14
    CRISPR: The Revolutionary Tool 14
    Applications in Medicine 15
    Ethical Considerations 15
    Future Outlook 16
Regenerative Medicine 17
    Principles of Regenerative Medicine 17
    Current Applications 18

- Promising Future 19
- Challenges and Ethical Considerations 19
- Nanomedicine 21
  - Principles of Nanomedicine 21
  - Current Applications 22
  - Challenges and Considerations 23
  - Future Outlook 23
- Microbiome Science: Unraveling the Secrets of Our Inner Ecosystem 25
  - Understanding the Human Microbiome 25
  - Personalized Medicine and Microbiome Profiling 26
  - Microbiome-Based Therapeutics 27
  - Challenges and Considerations 27
- Blockchain Technology in Healthcare 29
  - Understanding Blockchain Technology 29
  - Applications of Blockchain in Healthcare 29
  - Benefits of Blockchain in Healthcare 30
  - Challenges and Considerations 31
  - Future Outlook 32
- Bioinformatics and Genomics: Transforming Healthcare with Data 33
  - The Role of Bioinformatics in Genomics 33
  - Advancements in Genomics and Their Impact on Healthcare 34
  - Innovations in Bioinformatics and Genomics 35

- Challenges and Considerations 35
- Immunotherapy: Harnessing the Immune System for Advanced Treatments 37
  - The Basics of Immunotherapy 37
  - Advancements in Immunotherapy 38
  - Immunotherapy Beyond Cancer 39
  - Challenges and Considerations 39
- Mental Health Innovations: Revolutionizing Care for the Future 41
  - Teletherapy and Remote Mental Health Services 41
  - Digital Therapeutics and Apps 42
  - Wearable Technology and Mental Health Monitoring 43
  - Emerging Therapies and Treatments 43
  - Challenges and Considerations 44
- Precision Oncology: Tailoring Cancer Treatments for Individual Patients 45
  - Understanding Precision Oncology 45
  - Emerging Trends in Precision Oncology 46
  - Applications of Precision Oncology 47
  - Challenges and Considerations 47
- Nutrigenomics: Personalizing Nutrition Based on Genetic Makeup 49
  - Understanding Nutrigenomics 49
  - Emerging Trends in Nutrigenomics 50
  - Applications of Nutrigenomics 51
  - Challenges and Considerations 51

Bioprinting: The Future of Tissue and Organ Regeneration 53

    Understanding Bioprinting 53

    Emerging Trends in Bioprinting 54

    Applications of Bioprinting 55

    Challenges and Considerations 55

Smart Pill Bottles: Enhancing Medication Management 57

    Understanding Smart Pill Bottles 57

    Emerging Trends in Smart Pill Bottles 58

    Applications of Smart Pill Bottles 59

    Challenges and Considerations 59

Nanoscale Drug Delivery: Revolutionizing Targeted Therapy 61

    Understanding Nanoscale Drug Delivery 61

    Emerging Trends in Nanoscale Drug Delivery 62

    Applications of Nanoscale Drug Delivery 63

    Challenges and Considerations 63

Health Gamification: Revolutionizing Wellness and Treatment 65

    Understanding Health Gamification 65

    Emerging Trends in Health Gamification 66

    Applications of Health Gamification 67

    Challenges and Considerations 67

Drug Repurposing: Unlocking New Uses for Existing Medications 69

    Understanding Drug Repurposing 69

- Emerging Trends in Drug Repurposing 70
- Applications of Drug Repurposing 71
- Challenges and Considerations 71

Lab-on-a-Chip: Revolutionizing Diagnostics and Research 73
- Understanding Lab-on-a-Chip Technology 73
- Emerging Trends in Lab-on-a-Chip Technology 74
- Applications of Lab-on-a-Chip Technology 75
- Challenges and Considerations 75

Wearable Health Tech: The Future of Personal Health Monitoring 77
- Evolution of Wearable Health Tech 77
- Innovative Applications of Wearable Health Tech 78
- Integration with Healthcare Systems 79
- Future Trends in Wearable Health Tech 79
- Challenges and Considerations 80

glossary 81

Appendix 86
- A. Additional Resources 86
- B. Further Reading 87
- C. Supplementary Information 88

Disclaimer 90

8

INTRODUCTION TO FUTURISTIC CONCEPTS IN MEDICINE

The field of medicine has always been a dynamic and evolving discipline, continuously pushing the boundaries of what is possible. From the earliest days of healing practices rooted in natural remedies to the sophisticated techniques of modern surgery and pharmaceuticals, medicine has come a long way. However, we are now on the brink of a new era—one that promises to transform the landscape of healthcare as we know it. This chapter serves as an introduction to the cutting-edge advancements and futuristic concepts in medicine that are poised to revolutionize how we diagnose, treat, and manage health conditions.

THE MEDICAL FRONTIER

As technology advances at an unprecedented pace, the integration of these innovations into medical practices offers exciting opportunities to enhance patient care and improve outcomes. This convergence of technology and medicine encompasses a wide range of disciplines, from artificial intelligence (AI) and robotics to gene editing and regenerative medicine. These emerging fields hold the promise of more precise, personalized, and efficient healthcare delivery, addressing not only existing challenges but also paving the way for entirely new approaches to patient care.

THE POTENTIAL IMPACT

The impact of these futuristic concepts extends beyond the traditional confines of medicine. They have the potential to reshape the entire healthcare ecosystem, from the way medical professionals are trained and the tools they use, to how patients access care and the role of data in healthcare decision-making. As we explore these emerging technologies, we must also consider the ethical, regulatory, and societal implications that come with them.

A NEW AGE OF MEDICINE

The advent of advanced medical technologies marks the beginning of a new age in medicine— one that emphasizes prevention, precision, and personalization. The future of healthcare will be characterized by treatments tailored to individual genetic profiles, wearable devices that monitor health in real-time, and AI-driven diagnostics that can detect diseases at their earliest stages. This shift from a one-size-fits-all approach to a more tailored strategy holds the potential to drastically improve patient outcomes and quality of life.

CHALLENGES AND OPPORTUNITIES

While the potential benefits of these futuristic concepts are immense, there are also significant challenges to navigate. Ethical dilemmas arise when considering interventions such as gene editing, which could have far-reaching consequences for individuals and society at large. The use of AI in healthcare raises questions about the role of human judgment and the potential for bias in algorithms. Additionally, regulatory frameworks must evolve to keep pace with these rapid advancements, ensuring that new technologies are safe and accessible.

ARTIFICIAL INTELLIGENCE IN MEDICINE

Artificial Intelligence (AI) is one of the most transformative technologies impacting the field of medicine today. By leveraging machine learning algorithms, AI has the potential to revolutionize diagnostics, treatment planning, and medical research. In this chapter, we will explore the various applications of AI in healthcare and examine how it is changing the landscape of patient care.

AI-POWERED DIAGNOSTICS

AI is making significant strides in diagnostics, providing medical professionals with powerful tools to analyze medical images and data. Machine learning algorithms can be trained to recognize patterns and anomalies in medical images, such as X-rays, MRIs, and CT scans, with remarkable accuracy. These algorithms can assist radiologists in detecting diseases like cancer, fractures, and other conditions, often with a speed and precision that rivals or surpasses human experts.

For example, AI algorithms have been developed to identify early signs of breast cancer in mammograms, leading to earlier diagnoses and improved treatment outcomes. Similarly, AI-powered diagnostic tools have been applied to detect diabetic retinopathy, a condition that can lead to blindness if not caught early. By aiding in early detection, AI can help save lives and reduce the burden on healthcare systems.

AI-DRIVEN TREATMENT PLANNING

Beyond diagnostics, AI is also playing a key role in treatment planning. Personalized medicine, which tailors treatments to individual patients based on their genetic makeup and other factors, can benefit greatly from AI's ability to analyze large datasets. AI algorithms can process a patient's medical history, genetic information, and other data to recommend the most effective treatment options.

AI-driven treatment planning can also optimize the delivery of therapies such as radiation treatment for cancer. Algorithms can calculate the most precise dosage and positioning for radiation beams, maximizing the treatment's effectiveness while minimizing harm to healthy tissues.

MEDICAL RESEARCH AND DRUG DISCOVERY

AI's impact extends to medical research and drug discovery as well. By processing vast amounts of data from clinical trials and research studies, AI can identify patterns and correlations that may not be immediately apparent to human researchers. This can lead to new insights into disease mechanisms and potential treatment targets.

AI-driven drug discovery is another area of significant potential. Traditionally, the process of identifying and developing new drugs is time-consuming and expensive. AI can accelerate this process by screening vast libraries of compounds and predicting their potential efficacy against specific diseases. This can lead to the discovery of new drugs and treatments more quickly and cost-effectively.

AI IN PATIENT CARE

AI's role in patient care is not limited to diagnostics and treatment planning. Chatbots and virtual assistants powered by AI can provide patients with information and support, answering questions about their conditions and treatments. These tools can also help patients manage their health by providing reminders for medications and appointments.

In addition, AI can assist healthcare providers in making more informed decisions about patient care. By analyzing data from electronic health records, AI can identify trends and potential risks, helping doctors intervene earlier and provide more targeted care.

CHALLENGES AND ETHICAL CONSIDERATIONS

While AI offers immense potential in medicine, it also presents challenges and ethical considerations. One key concern is the potential for bias in AI algorithms, which could lead to disparities in healthcare outcomes. Ensuring that AI models are trained on diverse and representative datasets is crucial to mitigate this risk.

Another challenge is the potential for AI to impact the doctor-patient relationship. While AI can enhance medical decision-making, it should not replace the human touch and empathy that are integral to patient care.

GENE EDITING

Gene editing is a groundbreaking area of medical research that has the potential to revolutionize the way we understand and treat genetic diseases. The ability to modify an organism's DNA with precision offers a wide range of possibilities, from curing hereditary illnesses to enhancing crop resilience in agriculture. In this chapter, we will explore the most prominent gene editing technology, its applications in medicine, and the ethical considerations surrounding its use.

CRISPR: THE REVOLUTIONARY TOOL

CRISPR (Clustered Regularly Interspaced Short Palindromic Repeats) is a gene editing technology that has garnered significant attention due to its efficiency, versatility, and relatively low cost. This system, derived from a naturally occurring bacterial immune response, uses a guide RNA molecule to target specific DNA sequences. The Cas9 enzyme then creates a break in the DNA at the target site, allowing for the addition, deletion, or modification of genetic material.

CRISPR has transformed the field of gene editing by making it more accessible and precise. Its applications extend beyond research laboratories and into various industries, including agriculture, biotechnology, and medicine.

APPLICATIONS IN MEDICINE

Gene editing holds immense promise in the medical field, particularly in the treatment and prevention of genetic disorders. Some key areas of application include:

- Monogenic Diseases: CRISPR can potentially correct mutations that cause monogenic diseases, such as cystic fibrosis, sickle cell anemia, and muscular dystrophy. By targeting and repairing the specific genetic defects, gene editing offers a potential cure for these conditions.

- Cancer Therapy: Gene editing can be used to modify immune cells to target and destroy cancer cells more effectively. Chimeric antigen receptor (CAR) T-cell therapy, for example, involves engineering a patient's T-cells to recognize and attack cancer cells.

- Infectious Diseases: Gene editing may be used to develop treatments for infectious diseases by altering the host's genetic makeup to resist pathogens or by engineering pathogens themselves to be less virulent.

- Rare Diseases: For individuals with rare genetic disorders, gene editing may offer a lifeline by providing treatments that would otherwise be unavailable. Customizing therapies for these rare conditions can greatly improve patients' quality of life.

ETHICAL CONSIDERATIONS

While gene editing presents exciting possibilities, it also raises significant ethical concerns that must be carefully addressed. Some of the primary issues include:

- **Germline Editing**: Editing genes in reproductive cells can lead to heritable changes, which raises concerns about potential unintended consequences for future generations. Many countries have strict regulations against germline editing due to these risks.

- **Equity and Access**: As with any new medical technology, there is the risk of disparities in access to gene editing therapies. Ensuring equitable distribution and availability of treatments is crucial to avoid exacerbating existing healthcare inequalities.

- **Off-Target Effects**: Despite its precision, gene editing can sometimes cause unintended changes to DNA at sites other than the intended target. These off-target effects can lead to unknown risks and complications.

- **Designer Babies**: The possibility of using gene editing to select for specific traits in embryos, such as intelligence or physical appearance, raises ethical questions about the potential for creating "designer babies" and altering human diversity.

FUTURE OUTLOOK

Gene editing is a rapidly evolving field with immense potential to transform medicine and other industries. As researchers continue to advance the technology and address ethical concerns, gene editing may become a standard tool in medical practice. It could enable us to not only treat but potentially eliminate many genetic diseases, improving the quality of life for countless individuals.

REGENERATIVE MEDICINE

Regenerative medicine is a rapidly evolving field that seeks to restore and replace damaged tissues and organs using a combination of stem cell therapy, tissue engineering, and biomaterials. By harnessing the body's natural ability to heal and regenerate, regenerative medicine holds the potential to revolutionize how we treat a wide range of injuries and diseases. In this chapter, we will explore the principles of regenerative medicine, its current applications, and the promising future it offers.

PRINCIPLES OF REGENERATIVE MEDICINE

At its core, regenerative medicine aims to repair, replace, or regenerate damaged tissues and organs. This is achieved through the use of stem cells, biomaterials, and tissue engineering techniques. The key principles of regenerative medicine include:

- Stem Cell Therapy: Stem cells are undifferentiated cells that have the potential to develop into various specialized cell types. They can be harvested from sources such as bone marrow, adipose tissue, and umbilical cord blood. Stem cells can be used to regenerate damaged tissues and organs by differentiating into the desired cell types.

- Tissue Engineering: Tissue engineering involves combining cells, biomaterials, and signaling molecules to create functional tissues and organs in the lab. These engineered tissues can be used for transplantation or to study disease processes and drug responses.

- Biomaterials: Biomaterials play a crucial role in regenerative medicine by providing structural support and facilitating cell growth and differentiation. They can be natural or synthetic and are often designed to mimic the extracellular matrix of tissues.

CURRENT APPLICATIONS

Regenerative medicine has already made significant strides in several areas of medical practice. Some notable applications include:

- Wound Healing: Stem cell therapy and growth factors have been used to promote wound healing in patients with chronic ulcers and burns. These treatments can accelerate tissue repair and reduce the risk of infection.

- Orthopedics: Regenerative medicine is being used to treat musculoskeletal injuries, such as cartilage damage and bone fractures. Stem cells and tissue-engineered scaffolds can enhance the healing process and improve function.

- Cardiology: In the field of cardiology, stem cell therapy is being investigated for its potential to regenerate damaged heart tissue after a heart attack. This approach could improve heart function and reduce the risk of heart failure.

- Organ Transplants: Tissue engineering holds promise for creating lab-grown organs for transplantation, potentially addressing the shortage of donor organs. This would enable patients to receive transplants more quickly and with fewer complications.

PROMISING FUTURE

The future of regenerative medicine looks incredibly promising as researchers continue to advance the field. Some potential developments include:

- Personalized Medicine: Regenerative medicine may play a key role in personalized medicine by allowing treatments to be tailored to an individual's specific genetic makeup and medical history.

- 3D Bioprinting: 3D bioprinting is an emerging technology that enables the creation of complex tissues and organs using bio-inks and cells. This technique could revolutionize organ transplantation by providing a consistent and customizable supply of organs.

- Gene-Edited Therapies: Combining gene editing with regenerative medicine could lead to more precise and effective treatments. Gene-edited stem cells, for example, could be used to correct genetic defects and promote tissue regeneration.

CHALLENGES AND ETHICAL CONSIDERATIONS

While regenerative medicine offers immense potential, it also presents challenges and ethical considerations that must be addressed:

- Immune Rejection: Transplanted tissues and organs may be rejected by the recipient's immune system. Researchers are exploring ways to create immune-compatible tissues to reduce the risk of rejection.

- Ethical Concerns: The use of embryonic stem cells in research raises ethical concerns. Alternative sources, such as induced pluripotent stem cells (iPSCs), are being developed to address these issues.

- Regulation and Safety: Ensuring the safety and efficacy of regenerative medicine treatments is crucial. Regulatory agencies play a key role in overseeing the development and approval of these therapies.

NANOMEDICINE

Nanomedicine is an emerging field that leverages the unique properties of nanoparticles and nanoscale materials to diagnose, treat, and prevent diseases at the molecular level. This innovative approach offers the potential to revolutionize healthcare by providing more targeted and effective treatments with fewer side effects. In this chapter, we will explore the principles of nanomedicine, its current applications, and the challenges and opportunities it presents for the future of healthcare.

PRINCIPLES OF NANOMEDICINE

Nanomedicine involves the use of materials and devices at the nanoscale (typically 1 to 100 nanometers) to interact with biological systems. The small size of nanoparticles allows them to penetrate cells and tissues more effectively, providing opportunities for targeted drug delivery, advanced diagnostics, and other medical applications. Key principles of nanomedicine include:

- Targeted Drug Delivery: Nanoparticles can be engineered to carry drugs and other therapeutic agents directly to specific cells or tissues, minimizing the impact on healthy cells and reducing side effects.

- Diagnostics and Imaging: Nanoparticles can be designed to enhance imaging techniques, such as MRI and PET scans, making it easier to detect diseases at an earlier stage.

- Regenerative Medicine: Nanomaterials can be used to promote tissue regeneration and repair by providing scaffolds for cell growth and differentiation.

- Nanorobotics: In the future, nanorobots could be used for precise medical interventions, such as repairing damaged tissues or delivering drugs directly to diseased cells.

CURRENT APPLICATIONS

Nanomedicine is already making an impact in several areas of healthcare:

- Cancer Treatment: Nanoparticles can be used to deliver chemotherapy drugs directly to tumor cells, reducing the impact on healthy tissues and increasing the efficacy of treatment. Additionally, nanoparticles can be engineered to selectively destroy cancer cells through targeted thermal therapy.

- Drug Delivery: Nanoparticles can be used to deliver drugs more efficiently, improving absorption and bioavailability. This can lead to lower doses and reduced side effects.

- Imaging: Nanoparticles can be used as contrast agents in imaging techniques, such as MRI and CT scans, providing clearer and more detailed images for diagnostics.

- Vaccines: Nanotechnology has been used to develop novel vaccine delivery systems, improving the stability and efficacy of vaccines and enabling the development of new vaccines against emerging diseases.

CHALLENGES AND CONSIDERATIONS

Despite the potential of nanomedicine, there are challenges and considerations that must be addressed:

- Safety and Toxicity: The safety of nanoparticles is a major concern, as their small size can lead to unexpected interactions with biological systems. Rigorous testing and regulation are needed to ensure the safety of nanomedicine products.

- Regulation and Approval: Nanomedicine products face regulatory challenges due to their novel nature. Clear guidelines and standards are needed to facilitate the development and approval of nanomedicine therapies.

- Manufacturing and Scalability: Producing nanoparticles consistently and at scale can be challenging. Advances in manufacturing processes are necessary to bring nanomedicine products to market.

- Ethical and Social Implications: The use of nanotechnology in medicine raises ethical and social questions, such as potential misuse for enhancement purposes and concerns about environmental impact.

FUTURE OUTLOOK

The future of nanomedicine is promising, with ongoing research focused on improving the safety, efficacy, and scalability of nanotechnology-based therapies. Potential developments include:

- Nanorobotics: The use of nanorobots for targeted medical interventions could revolutionize surgery and other treatments.

- Personalized Medicine: Nanomedicine can play a key role in personalized medicine by enabling the delivery of customized treatments based on an individual's genetic profile.

- Nanotechnology in Regenerative Medicine: The integration of nanotechnology with regenerative medicine could lead to the development of more advanced tissue engineering techniques and regenerative therapies.

MICROBIOME SCIENCE: UNRAVELING THE SECRETS OF OUR INNER ECOSYSTEM

The human microbiome is a complex community of microorganisms—including bacteria, viruses, fungi, and other microbes—that live on and inside our bodies. This inner ecosystem plays a crucial role in our health, influencing everything from digestion and immunity to mood and metabolism. Advances in microbiome science are leading to a new era of personalized medicine and transformative healthcare approaches. In this chapter, we will explore the future of microbiome science and its potential impact on medical practice.

UNDERSTANDING THE HUMAN MICROBIOME

The human microbiome is a diverse and dynamic community of microorganisms that varies from person to person. It is most densely populated in the gut, but it is also present on the skin, in the mouth, and in other areas. Researchers have discovered that the microbiome influences a wide range of bodily functions, including:

- Digestion and Metabolism: The gut microbiome helps break down food and extract nutrients, influencing metabolism and weight management.

- Immunity: A healthy microbiome supports the immune system by defending against pathogens and regulating immune responses.

- Brain Function: Emerging research suggests that the gut-brain axis connects the microbiome with brain function, affecting mood, behavior, and cognitive health.

- Chronic Diseases: An imbalance in the microbiome, known as dysbiosis, has been linked to chronic diseases such as diabetes, inflammatory bowel disease (IBD), and obesity.

PERSONALIZED MEDICINE AND MICROBIOME PROFILING

Advances in microbiome science are enabling more personalized approaches to healthcare:

- Microbiome Sequencing: High-throughput sequencing techniques allow for detailed profiling of an individual's microbiome. This information can guide personalized treatment plans and dietary recommendations.

- Targeted Probiotics: Researchers are developing targeted probiotics tailored to an individual's microbiome to restore balance and support health.

- Microbiome Modulation: Strategies to modulate the microbiome, such as fecal microbiota transplantation (FMT), are being explored to treat conditions like Clostridioides difficile infection and IBD.

- Precision Nutrition: Understanding an individual's microbiome can inform personalized dietary recommendations to optimize health and prevent disease.

MICROBIOME-BASED THERAPEUTICS

Microbiome science is paving the way for innovative therapeutic approaches:

- Live Biotherapeutics: Live biotherapeutics are products containing live microbes that can modulate the microbiome to treat diseases. For example, certain strains of bacteria are being investigated as treatments for gastrointestinal disorders.

- Microbial Metabolites: Microbes produce metabolites that can influence health. Researchers are exploring the therapeutic potential of these metabolites for conditions such as cancer and metabolic disorders.

- Bacteriophage Therapy: Bacteriophages, or viruses that infect bacteria, can be used to target specific harmful bacteria without disrupting the overall microbiome.

CHALLENGES AND CONSIDERATIONS

While microbiome science holds great promise, there are challenges and considerations to address:

- Complexity and Variability: The microbiome is highly complex and varies widely among individuals, making it challenging to develop standardized treatments.

- Ethical and Regulatory Issues: Research involving microbiome manipulation must address ethical and regulatory concerns, including safety and informed consent.

- Data Privacy: Protecting the privacy of microbiome data is essential, as it can reveal sensitive information about an individual's health.

- Long-Term Effects: The long-term effects of microbiome interventions are still not fully understood, and careful monitoring is needed.

BLOCKCHAIN TECHNOLOGY IN HEALTHCARE

Blockchain technology is gaining attention in the healthcare industry as a secure, decentralized method for managing data and transactions. By providing a transparent and tamper-proof ledger, blockchain has the potential to enhance data security, interoperability, and efficiency in healthcare. In this chapter, we will explore the applications of blockchain technology in healthcare, its benefits, and the challenges it presents.

UNDERSTANDING BLOCKCHAIN TECHNOLOGY

Blockchain is a distributed ledger technology that records transactions across multiple computers in a secure and transparent manner. Each transaction, or block, is linked to the previous one, forming a chain. The decentralized nature of blockchain ensures that data is secure, tamper-proof, and verifiable.

APPLICATIONS OF BLOCKCHAIN IN HEALTHCARE

Blockchain technology has various applications in healthcare, including:

- Electronic Health Records (EHRs): Blockchain can provide a secure and interoperable system for managing and sharing EHRs across different healthcare providers. Patients can control access to their data and grant permissions to specific providers.

- Supply Chain Management: Blockchain can enhance transparency and traceability in the healthcare supply chain, ensuring the authenticity of medical products and reducing the risk of counterfeit drugs.

- Clinical Trials and Research: Blockchain can improve the integrity and transparency of clinical trials by securely recording data and ensuring that it cannot be altered. This can increase trust in research results and streamline the approval process.

- Insurance Claims Processing: Blockchain can automate and expedite insurance claims processing by securely verifying patient data and medical records, reducing fraud and administrative costs.

- Data Sharing and Consent Management: Blockchain can enable secure and efficient data sharing among healthcare providers, researchers, and patients. Patients can manage their data and provide informed consent for its use in research.

BENEFITS OF BLOCKCHAIN IN HEALTHCARE

Blockchain offers several benefits for the healthcare industry:

- Data Security and Integrity: Blockchain's decentralized and encrypted ledger ensures the security and integrity of healthcare data, reducing the risk of data breaches and fraud.

- Interoperability: Blockchain can facilitate data interoperability across different healthcare systems and providers, improving the flow of information and enhancing patient care.

- Patient Empowerment: Blockchain allows patients to have more control over their health data and manage access permissions, empowering them to be active participants in their healthcare.

- Efficiency and Cost Savings: Blockchain can streamline administrative processes, such as insurance claims and data sharing, reducing costs and improving efficiency.

CHALLENGES AND CONSIDERATIONS

While blockchain technology offers many benefits, there are challenges and considerations to address:

- Regulatory and Legal Issues: The use of blockchain in healthcare raises regulatory and legal questions, such as compliance with data protection laws and the legal recognition of blockchain records.

- Scalability and Performance: The scalability and performance of blockchain networks can be limited, especially as the size of the network and the volume of transactions increase.

- Standardization and Adoption: Standardization of blockchain protocols and widespread adoption are necessary for its effective implementation in healthcare.

- Technical Complexity: The complexity of blockchain technology can be a barrier to its adoption, requiring specialized knowledge and training for healthcare professionals.

FUTURE OUTLOOK

The future of blockchain in healthcare is promising, with potential developments including:

- Integration with Emerging Technologies: Combining blockchain with other technologies such as AI and IoT can enhance its applications in healthcare and create new opportunities.

- Global Health Data Networks: Blockchain can enable the creation of secure and interoperable global health data networks, facilitating research and improving patient care worldwide.

- Decentralized Health Platforms: Blockchain can support the development of decentralized health platforms where patients can securely manage their health data and access healthcare services.

BIOINFORMATICS AND GENOMICS: TRANSFORMING HEALTHCARE WITH DATA

Bioinformatics and genomics are interdisciplinary fields that leverage computational tools to analyze and interpret biological data, particularly genetic and genomic information. These disciplines are revolutionizing healthcare by enabling personalized medicine, improving diagnostics, and advancing our understanding of diseases. In this chapter, we will explore the future of bioinformatics and genomics, highlighting emerging trends and concrete examples of how they are shaping the healthcare landscape.

THE ROLE OF BIOINFORMATICS IN GENOMICS

Bioinformatics is the application of computational methods to manage, analyze, and interpret biological data. In genomics, bioinformatics plays a crucial role in processing large datasets and extracting meaningful insights. Some key areas where bioinformatics and genomics intersect include:

- Genome Sequencing: Bioinformatics is essential for analyzing high-throughput sequencing data, assembling genomes, and identifying genetic variants.

- Functional Genomics: This area involves studying the function of genes and their interactions using bioinformatics tools such as gene expression analysis and pathway modeling.

- Comparative Genomics: Bioinformatics enables the comparison of genomes across species, providing insights into evolution and the conservation of genetic elements.

- Proteomics and Metabolomics: These fields study proteins and metabolites, respectively, using bioinformatics to analyze complex datasets and identify patterns.

ADVANCEMENTS IN GENOMICS AND THEIR IMPACT ON HEALTHCARE

Genomics is driving transformative changes in healthcare, including:

- Precision Medicine: Genomic data allows for personalized treatment plans tailored to an individual's genetic makeup. For example, targeted therapies for cancer can be designed based on specific genetic mutations.

- Genomic Screening: Genome-wide screening can identify genetic predispositions to diseases, enabling early interventions and preventive measures.

- Pharmacogenomics: Understanding how genes affect an individual's response to medications allows for personalized prescribing and reduces the risk of adverse drug reactions.

- Gene Editing: Technologies like CRISPR have the potential to treat genetic disorders by precisely editing DNA sequences.

INNOVATIONS IN BIOINFORMATICS AND GENOMICS

Emerging trends in bioinformatics and genomics are driving innovation in healthcare:

- Machine Learning: Machine learning algorithms are being used to analyze complex genomic data and predict disease risk, treatment response, and patient outcomes.

- Population Genomics: Large-scale genomic studies of diverse populations provide insights into genetic variations and their impact on health and disease.

- Synthetic Biology: Bioinformatics is integral to designing and engineering new genetic sequences and organisms for medical applications.

- Real-Time Genomic Surveillance: Bioinformatics tools can monitor and track genetic changes in pathogens, aiding in the detection and response to infectious disease outbreaks.

CHALLENGES AND CONSIDERATIONS

Despite the potential of bioinformatics and genomics, there are challenges and considerations to address:

- Data Privacy and Security: Protecting the privacy of genomic data is crucial, as it can reveal sensitive information about an individual's health and identity.

- Data Interpretation: Analyzing and interpreting complex genomic data requires expertise, and there is a risk of misinterpretation.

- Ethical and Regulatory Issues: Ethical considerations include the potential for genetic discrimination and the need for informed consent in genomic research.

- Access and Equity: Ensuring equitable access to genomic medicine and data resources is essential for diverse and inclusive healthcare.

IMMUNOTHERAPY: HARNESSING THE IMMUNE SYSTEM FOR ADVANCED TREATMENTS

Immunotherapy is a groundbreaking approach to treating diseases by harnessing the power of the immune system. This innovative method has shown particular promise in oncology, where it has become a key tool for targeting and eradicating cancer cells. In this chapter, we will explore the future of immunotherapy, highlighting emerging trends and concrete examples of how it is revolutionizing healthcare.

THE BASICS OF IMMUNOTHERAPY

Immunotherapy leverages the body's immune system to fight diseases, particularly cancer. This approach includes various strategies:

- Checkpoint Inhibitors: These drugs block proteins that prevent the immune system from attacking cancer cells. By inhibiting these checkpoints, the immune system can recognize and destroy cancer cells.

- CAR-T Cell Therapy: Chimeric antigen receptor T-cell (CAR-T) therapy involves engineering a patient's T cells to recognize and attack specific cancer cells. These modified cells are then infused back into the patient.

- Cancer Vaccines: Cancer vaccines stimulate the immune system to recognize and attack cancer cells. Some vaccines target specific cancer antigens, while others use the patient's own tumor cells to create a personalized vaccine.

- Monoclonal Antibodies: These lab-created antibodies bind to specific targets on cancer cells or immune cells, enhancing the immune response or directly attacking the cancer.

ADVANCEMENTS IN IMMUNOTHERAPY

Immunotherapy is continuously evolving, with exciting advancements on the horizon:

- Bispecific Antibodies: These antibodies can bind to two different targets simultaneously, bringing cancer cells and immune cells closer together to enhance the immune response.

- Oncolytic Virus Therapy: Oncolytic viruses are engineered to selectively infect and kill cancer cells while stimulating an immune response against the tumor.

- Neoantigen Vaccines: These personalized vaccines target unique antigens found in an individual's tumor, prompting a targeted immune response.

- Combination Therapies: Combining immunotherapy with other treatments, such as chemotherapy or targeted therapy, can enhance efficacy and overcome resistance.

IMMUNOTHERAPY BEYOND CANCER

While immunotherapy has been most successful in treating cancer, it is also being explored for other conditions:

- Autoimmune Diseases: Researchers are investigating ways to use immunotherapy to modulate the immune system and treat autoimmune conditions such as rheumatoid arthritis and multiple sclerosis.

- Infectious Diseases: Immunotherapy approaches are being explored for treating viral infections, including potential therapies for diseases like HIV and COVID-19.

- Allergies: Immunotherapy is being used to desensitize individuals to allergens and reduce allergic reactions.

CHALLENGES AND CONSIDERATIONS

Despite its potential, immunotherapy presents challenges and considerations:

- Adverse Effects: Immunotherapy can cause immune-related side effects, including inflammation and autoimmune reactions.

- Cost and Access: Immunotherapies can be expensive, and ensuring equitable access to these treatments is important.

- Resistance and Relapse: Cancer cells can develop resistance to immunotherapy, leading to potential relapse.

- Precision Medicine: Identifying the right patients and tailoring immunotherapy treatments to their unique genetic profiles is key to maximizing effectiveness.

MENTAL HEALTH INNOVATIONS: REVOLUTIONIZING CARE FOR THE FUTURE

Mental health care has undergone significant changes in recent years, driven by technological advancements and an increased understanding of the complexities of mental health conditions. Innovations in this field are paving the way for more personalized, accessible, and effective treatments. In this chapter, we will explore the future of mental health care, highlighting emerging trends and concrete examples of how these innovations are transforming the landscape.

TELETHERAPY AND REMOTE MENTAL HEALTH SERVICES

Teletherapy and remote mental health services have become increasingly popular, providing convenient and accessible care to individuals worldwide:

- Video and Phone Counseling: Teletherapy enables individuals to receive counseling and therapy sessions through video or phone calls, reducing barriers such as travel time and location.

- Online Support Groups: Virtual support groups allow individuals to connect with others facing similar challenges, offering a sense of community and understanding.

- AI-Powered Chatbots: AI-driven chatbots provide immediate, confidential support and resources for individuals experiencing emotional distress.

DIGITAL THERAPEUTICS AND APPS

Digital therapeutics and mental health apps offer innovative tools for self-management and treatment:

- Cognitive Behavioral Therapy (CBT) Apps: Apps that deliver CBT interventions help individuals manage anxiety, depression, and other conditions through structured exercises.

- Mood Tracking and Journaling: Apps allow individuals to track their moods, emotions, and triggers, providing insights for managing their mental health.

- Meditation and Mindfulness Apps: Guided meditation and mindfulness exercises can reduce stress and improve overall well-being.

- Sleep Monitoring and Improvement: Apps that monitor sleep patterns and provide tips for better sleep contribute to improved mental health.

WEARABLE TECHNOLOGY AND MENTAL HEALTH MONITORING

Wearable devices are being used to monitor mental health and offer personalized interventions:

- Stress and Anxiety Detection: Wearables with sensors can detect physiological indicators of stress and anxiety, providing real-time feedback and coping strategies.
- Sleep and Activity Tracking: Wearables monitor sleep quality and activity levels, offering insights into how these factors impact mental health.
- Emotion Recognition: Advanced wearables may use facial recognition and voice analysis to assess emotional states and provide tailored support.

EMERGING THERAPIES AND TREATMENTS

New therapies and treatments are being explored to address mental health conditions:

- Transcranial Magnetic Stimulation (TMS): TMS is a non-invasive treatment that uses magnetic fields to stimulate specific areas of the brain, helping alleviate symptoms of depression.

- Ketamine-Assisted Therapy: Ketamine therapy, combined with counseling, shows promise in treating severe depression and post-traumatic stress disorder (PTSD).

- Psychedelic Therapies: Substances like psilocybin and MDMA are being studied for their potential to treat depression, anxiety, and PTSD in controlled therapeutic settings.

CHALLENGES AND CONSIDERATIONS

While mental health innovations offer many benefits, there are challenges and considerations to address:

- Accessibility and Equity: Ensuring equitable access to digital mental health tools and innovative therapies is essential for inclusive care.

- Data Privacy and Security: Protecting the privacy of mental health data collected through apps and wearables is crucial.

- Stigma and Acceptance: Reducing stigma around mental health and acceptance of new therapies remains a challenge.

- Ethical and Regulatory Issues: Research involving emerging therapies such as psychedelics must address ethical and regulatory concerns.

PRECISION ONCOLOGY: TAILORING CANCER TREATMENTS FOR INDIVIDUAL PATIENTS

Precision oncology is revolutionizing cancer treatment by tailoring therapies to the unique genetic and molecular characteristics of each patient's tumor. This personalized approach improves treatment outcomes and minimizes side effects, offering new hope to individuals with cancer. In this chapter, we will explore the future of precision oncology, highlighting emerging trends and concrete examples of how this field is transforming cancer care.

UNDERSTANDING PRECISION ONCOLOGY

Precision oncology, also known as personalized or individualized cancer treatment, involves the use of genetic and molecular data to guide therapy decisions:

- Genetic Profiling: Analyzing the genetic makeup of a patient's tumor to identify specific mutations or abnormalities that drive cancer growth.

- Targeted Therapies: Developing drugs that target specific genetic mutations or molecular pathways unique to a patient's tumor.

- Biomarker Testing: Using biomarkers, such as proteins or other molecules, to predict a patient's response to a particular treatment.

- Immunotherapy: Harnessing the body's immune system to fight cancer, often informed by the tumor's genetic profile.

EMERGING TRENDS IN PRECISION ONCOLOGY

Several trends are shaping the future of precision oncology:

- Liquid Biopsies: Non-invasive tests that analyze circulating tumor cells or DNA in the blood, providing insights into a patient's cancer without the need for a tissue biopsy.

- AI and Machine Learning: Leveraging AI and machine learning to analyze complex genetic data and identify the most effective treatments for each patient.

- Combination Therapies: Combining targeted therapies and immunotherapies to improve treatment efficacy and reduce resistance.

- Cancer Vaccines: Developing personalized cancer vaccines based on a patient's tumor antigens to stimulate an immune response.

- Real-Time Monitoring: Using wearable devices and other technologies to monitor patients' responses to treatment and adjust therapies as needed.

APPLICATIONS OF PRECISION ONCOLOGY

Precision oncology is transforming various aspects of cancer care:

- Early Detection and Screening: Identifying individuals at high risk of cancer through genetic testing and targeted screening programs.

- Treatment Selection: Matching patients with the most effective targeted therapies based on their tumor's genetic profile.

- Disease Monitoring: Using liquid biopsies and other methods to track cancer progression and treatment response.

- Rare and Aggressive Cancers: Precision oncology offers new options for patients with rare or aggressive cancers that may not respond to traditional treatments.

- Clinical Trials: Designing clinical trials that focus on specific genetic mutations, making it easier to find effective treatments for patients.

CHALLENGES AND CONSIDERATIONS

As precision oncology advances, there are challenges and considerations to address:

- Access and Affordability: Ensuring equitable access to precision oncology treatments and genetic testing for all patients.

- Data Privacy and Security: Protecting patient data from unauthorized access and misuse, especially with genetic information.

- Regulation and Standards: Developing clear regulatory frameworks and standards for genetic testing and targeted therapies.

- Ethical Concerns: Addressing ethical issues such as informed consent and potential discrimination based on genetic information.

NUTRIGENOMICS: PERSONALIZING NUTRITION BASED ON GENETIC MAKEUP

Nutrigenomics is the study of how an individual's genetic makeup influences their response to nutrients and dietary components. This emerging field seeks to provide personalized nutrition recommendations based on a person's unique genetic profile, optimizing health outcomes and potentially preventing chronic diseases. In this chapter, we will explore the future of nutrigenomics, highlighting emerging trends and concrete examples of how this field is transforming nutrition and healthcare.

UNDERSTANDING NUTRIGENOMICS

Nutrigenomics combines nutrition science with genomics to understand how diet interacts with an individual's genetic variations:

- Genetic Profiling: Analyzing an individual's genetic code to identify specific gene variants related to nutrient metabolism and absorption.

- Personalized Diet Plans: Tailoring dietary recommendations to an individual's genetic profile to optimize nutrient intake and support overall health.

• Nutrient-Gene Interactions: Understanding how different nutrients interact with specific genes and how this impacts health outcomes.

• Nutritional Biomarkers: Identifying biomarkers that indicate an individual's nutritional status and response to dietary changes.

EMERGING TRENDS IN NUTRIGENOMICS

Several trends are shaping the future of nutrigenomics:

• At-Home Genetic Testing: Direct-to-consumer genetic testing kits are making it easier for individuals to access their genetic information and learn about their nutritional needs.

• AI and Big Data: Leveraging AI and big data to analyze complex genetic and dietary data, providing more accurate and actionable insights for personalized nutrition.

• Microbiome Integration: Combining microbiome analysis with genetic data to create more comprehensive and tailored dietary recommendations.

• Nutrigenomic Apps: Developing mobile apps that provide personalized nutrition guidance based on genetic data and food preferences.

• Nutrigenomic Research: Advancing research in nutrigenomics to identify new nutrient-gene interactions and their impact on health.

APPLICATIONS OF NUTRIGENOMICS

Nutrigenomics is transforming various aspects of nutrition and healthcare:

- Personalized Nutrition Plans: Creating tailored diet plans that consider an individual's genetic profile, lifestyle, and health goals.

- Weight Management: Designing weight management strategies based on genetic variations that affect metabolism and appetite.

- Disease Prevention: Identifying genetic risk factors for chronic diseases and recommending dietary changes to mitigate these risks.

- Sports Nutrition: Providing athletes with personalized nutrition plans to enhance performance and recovery based on their genetic makeup.

- Prenatal Nutrition: Offering nutrition recommendations for expecting mothers based on their genetic profiles to support healthy pregnancies.

CHALLENGES AND CONSIDERATIONS

As nutrigenomics advances, there are challenges and considerations to address:

- Data Privacy and Security: Protecting genetic and dietary data from unauthorized access and misuse.

- Accessibility and Affordability: Ensuring equitable access to nutrigenomics services for individuals across different socioeconomic backgrounds.

- Ethical Concerns: Addressing ethical issues such as informed consent and potential discrimination based on genetic information.

- Regulation and Standardization: Developing clear guidelines and standards for nutrigenomics testing and recommendations.

BIOPRINTING: THE FUTURE OF TISSUE AND ORGAN REGENERATION

Bioprinting is a revolutionary technology that uses 3D printing techniques to create living tissues and organs. This emerging field has the potential to transform healthcare by enabling the creation of customized tissues for medical research, drug testing, and ultimately, organ transplants. In this chapter, we will explore the future of bioprinting, highlighting emerging trends and concrete examples of how this field is shaping the future of medicine.

UNDERSTANDING BIOPRINTING

Bioprinting involves the layer-by-layer deposition of bio-inks—mixtures of living cells, growth factors, and other biomaterials—to create complex tissues and structures:

- Bio-inks: Specialized inks composed of living cells and other biomaterials used in the bioprinting process.

- Layered Printing: Building tissues layer by layer using advanced 3D printing technologies.

- Tissue Engineering: Combining cells, biomaterials, and bioprinting techniques to engineer functional tissues.

- Organ Regeneration: Exploring the potential to print fully functional organs for transplantation.

EMERGING TRENDS IN BIOPRINTING

Several trends are shaping the future of bioprinting:

- Advanced Bio-inks: Developing new bio-inks with improved cell compatibility and functionality to create complex tissues.

- Vascularization: Integrating blood vessels into printed tissues to ensure proper nutrient and oxygen delivery.

- Organ-on-a-Chip: Creating small, functional organ models on microchips for drug testing and medical research.

- Custom Prosthetics: Bioprinting customized prosthetics and implants that precisely match a patient's anatomy.

- Regenerative Medicine: Exploring the potential for bioprinting to regenerate damaged tissues and organs.

APPLICATIONS OF BIOPRINTING

Bioprinting is transforming various aspects of medicine and healthcare:

- Drug Testing and Development: Using printed tissues to test the safety and efficacy of new drugs, reducing reliance on animal testing.

- Disease Modeling: Creating tissue models to study diseases and develop targeted treatments.

- Organ Transplants: Investigating the potential to bioprint functional organs for transplantation, addressing the shortage of donor organs.

- Cosmetic and Reconstructive Surgery: Bioprinting tissues for reconstructive surgeries, such as skin grafts and cartilage repairs.

- Educational and Research Tools: Providing students and researchers with bioprinted tissues for educational purposes and scientific research.

CHALLENGES AND CONSIDERATIONS

As bioprinting advances, there are challenges and considerations to address:

- Technical Limitations: Overcoming challenges related to tissue complexity, vascularization, and the integration of printed tissues with the body.

- Regulation and Standardization: Developing clear regulatory frameworks and standards for bioprinting to ensure safety and efficacy.

- Ethical Concerns: Addressing ethical issues such as the potential for creating human-animal hybrid tissues and the use of bioprinting for non-medical purposes.

- Cost and Accessibility: Ensuring that bioprinting technologies are accessible and affordable for healthcare providers and patients.

SMART PILL BOTTLES: ENHANCING MEDICATION MANAGEMENT

Smart pill bottles are an innovative technology designed to help patients manage their medications more effectively. These high-tech devices incorporate various features such as reminders, tracking, and connectivity to support patients in adhering to their prescribed medication regimens. In this chapter, we will explore the future of smart pill bottles, highlighting emerging trends and concrete examples of how these devices are transforming medication management and patient care.

UNDERSTANDING SMART PILL BOTTLES

Smart pill bottles are designed to improve medication adherence and support patients in managing their prescriptions:

- Medication Reminders: Integrated alarms or notifications that remind patients when to take their medication.

- Tracking and Monitoring: Sensors and connectivity that track when and how much medication is taken.

- Connectivity: Integration with smartphones and other devices to provide real-time data and communication with healthcare providers.

- Dosage Management: Features that help measure and dispense the correct dosage of medication.

- Safety and Security: Mechanisms such as child-resistant caps and secure locks to prevent accidental ingestion.

EMERGING TRENDS IN SMART PILL BOTTLES

Several trends are shaping the future of smart pill bottles:

- AI and Machine Learning: Utilizing AI and machine learning to analyze patient data and predict potential issues with medication adherence.

- Voice Assistants: Integrating voice-activated assistants to provide hands-free medication management and support.

- Biometric Identification: Using biometric sensors, such as fingerprint recognition, to ensure the right patient takes the medication.

- Smart Packaging: Developing innovative packaging that protects medications and extends shelf life while providing data about storage conditions.

- Remote Monitoring: Connecting smart pill bottles to healthcare providers for real-time monitoring and support.

APPLICATIONS OF SMART PILL BOTTLES

Smart pill bottles are transforming various aspects of medication management and healthcare:

- Improved Adherence: Helping patients take their medications as prescribed, which can lead to better health outcomes.

- Chronic Disease Management: Supporting patients with chronic conditions such as diabetes or hypertension in managing their medications.

- Clinical Trials: Facilitating patient adherence and data collection in clinical trials, improving the quality of research.

- Elderly Care: Assisting older adults in managing multiple medications and reducing the risk of medication errors.

- Remote Patient Monitoring: Providing healthcare providers with data on patient medication use, enabling more personalized care.

CHALLENGES AND CONSIDERATIONS

As smart pill bottles advance, there are challenges and considerations to address:

- Privacy and Data Security: Ensuring patient data is protected and secure, particularly with connectivity features.

- Accessibility and Cost: Making smart pill bottles affordable and accessible to a wide range of patients.

- Integration with Healthcare Systems: Ensuring smart pill bottles can integrate seamlessly with electronic health records and other healthcare technologies.

- User Experience: Designing devices that are user-friendly and easy to use for all patients, including those with limited technology experience.

NANOSCALE DRUG DELIVERY: REVOLUTIONIZING TARGETED THERAPY

Nanoscale drug delivery is a cutting-edge technology that uses nanoparticles to deliver drugs precisely to targeted cells and tissues in the body. This approach enhances the efficacy of treatments while minimizing side effects, as it allows for controlled release and specific targeting of therapeutic agents. In this chapter, we will explore the future of nanoscale drug delivery, highlighting emerging trends and concrete examples of how this technology is transforming medicine.

UNDERSTANDING NANOSCALE DRUG DELIVERY

Nanoscale drug delivery involves the use of particles at the nanometer scale to transport drugs:

- Nanoparticles: Tiny particles, often between 1 and 100 nanometers in size, that can carry drugs to specific targets in the body.
- Targeted Therapy: Designing nanoparticles to target specific cells or tissues, such as cancer cells, while sparing healthy cells.

- Controlled Release: Engineering nanoparticles to release drugs at a controlled rate, optimizing treatment effectiveness.

- Biocompatibility: Ensuring nanoparticles are safe and compatible with the body's natural systems.

- Functionalization: Modifying the surface of nanoparticles to enhance targeting and delivery capabilities.

EMERGING TRENDS IN NANOSCALE DRUG DELIVERY

Several trends are shaping the future of nanoscale drug delivery:

- Smart Nanoparticles: Developing nanoparticles that respond to specific stimuli such as pH, temperature, or enzymes for controlled drug release.

- Multifunctional Nanoparticles: Creating nanoparticles that can deliver drugs, imaging agents, and other therapeutic compounds simultaneously.

- Personalized Nanomedicine: Tailoring nanoparticles to an individual's genetic and biological profile for optimized treatment.

- Nanocarrier Platforms: Designing versatile platforms for delivering a wide range of drugs, from small molecules to biologics.

• Nanotechnology in Vaccines: Using nanoparticles to enhance vaccine delivery and effectiveness.

APPLICATIONS OF NANOSCALE DRUG DELIVERY

Nanoscale drug delivery is transforming various aspects of medicine and healthcare:

• Cancer Treatment: Targeting tumors with nanoparticles that deliver chemotherapy directly to cancer cells, reducing side effects.

• Infectious Diseases: Enhancing the delivery of antibiotics and antiviral drugs to specific sites of infection.

• Neurological Disorders: Delivering drugs across the blood-brain barrier to treat conditions such as Alzheimer's and Parkinson's.

• Chronic Conditions: Providing sustained release of drugs for managing chronic conditions such as diabetes and arthritis.

• Gene Therapy: Utilizing nanoparticles to deliver genetic material for gene therapy applications.

CHALLENGES AND CONSIDERATIONS

As nanoscale drug delivery advances, there are challenges and considerations to address:

- Safety and Toxicity: Ensuring nanoparticles are safe for patients and do not cause unintended toxicity.

- Regulation and Standardization: Establishing clear guidelines and standards for the use of nanomaterials in medicine.

- Manufacturing and Scalability: Developing scalable manufacturing processes for the production of nanoparticles.

- Ethical Concerns: Addressing ethical issues related to the use of nanotechnology in medicine.

- Patient Acceptance: Educating patients and healthcare providers about the benefits and safety of nanoscale drug delivery.

HEALTH GAMIFICATION: REVOLUTIONIZING WELLNESS AND TREATMENT

Health gamification is the application of game design elements to health and wellness practices to engage and motivate individuals to achieve their health goals. By transforming aspects of healthcare into engaging and rewarding experiences, gamification encourages behavior change and enhances adherence to treatment plans. In this chapter, we will explore the future of health gamification, highlighting emerging trends and concrete examples of how it is transforming wellness and treatment.

UNDERSTANDING HEALTH GAMIFICATION

Health gamification integrates game-like elements into health and wellness activities to increase motivation and engagement:

- Points and Rewards: Offering points or rewards for completing health-related tasks such as exercise, medication adherence, or healthy eating.

- Challenges and Quests: Creating quests or challenges that encourage users to reach specific health goals.

• Progress Tracking: Providing visual representations of progress to keep users motivated and focused on their goals.

• Social Interaction: Enabling social features such as leaderboards and group challenges to foster a sense of community and competition.

• Virtual Reality (VR): Using VR to create immersive and interactive health and wellness experiences.

EMERGING TRENDS IN HEALTH GAMIFICATION

Several trends are shaping the future of health gamification:

• Personalization: Tailoring gamification elements to an individual's preferences, needs, and health goals for a more engaging experience.

• Integration with Wearables: Connecting gamification apps to wearable devices to track health metrics and provide real-time feedback.

• AI-Driven Gamification: Leveraging AI to analyze user data and provide personalized recommendations and challenges.

• Immersive Experiences: Developing VR and augmented reality (AR) experiences that make health activities more engaging.

• Therapeutic Gaming: Using video games and gamified apps as therapeutic tools for mental health and rehabilitation.

APPLICATIONS OF HEALTH GAMIFICATION

Health gamification is transforming various aspects of wellness and healthcare:

- Fitness and Exercise: Using apps and devices that turn exercise into a game, encouraging consistent physical activity.

- Nutrition and Diet: Offering gamified apps that reward healthy eating habits and provide nutritional guidance.

- Medication Adherence: Using gamification to remind and motivate patients to take their medications as prescribed.

- Chronic Disease Management: Helping patients with chronic conditions such as diabetes or hypertension manage their health through gamified tools.

- Mental Health Support: Providing interactive and engaging apps that offer cognitive behavioral therapy (CBT) and stress management techniques.

CHALLENGES AND CONSIDERATIONS

As health gamification advances, there are challenges and considerations to address:

- User Engagement: Ensuring gamified experiences remain engaging and motivating over time.

- Privacy and Data Security: Protecting user data and ensuring secure communication within gamified health platforms.

- Inclusivity and Accessibility: Designing gamified tools that are accessible and inclusive for all users, regardless of abilities or background.

- Efficacy and Safety: Verifying the efficacy and safety of gamified health interventions through research and clinical trials.

- Ethical Considerations: Addressing potential ethical concerns related to using game elements in healthcare.

DRUG REPURPOSING: UNLOCKING NEW USES FOR EXISTING MEDICATIONS

Drug repurposing, also known as drug repositioning, is the practice of finding new uses for existing medications beyond their original indications. This innovative approach leverages established drugs to treat different conditions, offering a faster and more cost-effective path to new therapies. In this chapter, we will explore the future of drug repurposing, highlighting emerging trends and concrete examples of how this strategy is revolutionizing the development of new treatments.

UNDERSTANDING DRUG REPURPOSING

Drug repurposing involves identifying alternative uses for approved drugs:

- Mechanism of Action: Investigating how a drug works in the body and exploring other conditions that could benefit from the same mechanism.

- Clinical Data Analysis: Examining existing clinical data to identify patterns or indications of a drug's potential efficacy for other conditions.

- Computational Approaches: Utilizing AI and machine learning to analyze large datasets and predict new uses for existing drugs.

- Safety Profile: Taking advantage of the established safety profile of existing drugs to accelerate the development process.

- Combination Therapy: Exploring potential combinations of repurposed drugs with other medications for synergistic effects.

EMERGING TRENDS IN DRUG REPURPOSING

Several trends are shaping the future of drug repurposing:

- AI and Machine Learning: Leveraging AI and machine learning algorithms to analyze large datasets and identify potential new uses for existing drugs.

- Data Sharing Initiatives: Collaborative efforts to share clinical data and research findings, facilitating the discovery of new drug uses.

- High-Throughput Screening: Utilizing automated screening methods to quickly test existing drugs against a range of targets.

- Precision Medicine: Combining drug repurposing with precision medicine approaches to tailor treatments to individual patients' genetic and molecular profiles.

- Crowdsourcing and Open Innovation: Engaging researchers, clinicians, and the public in identifying potential new uses for existing drugs.

APPLICATIONS OF DRUG REPURPOSING

Drug repurposing is transforming various aspects of healthcare and medicine:

- Cancer Treatment: Identifying existing drugs that can inhibit cancer growth or enhance the effectiveness of other treatments.
- Infectious Diseases: Discovering drugs that can target viruses, bacteria, or other pathogens, especially important during pandemics.
- Neurological Disorders: Exploring the potential of existing drugs to treat conditions such as Alzheimer's, Parkinson's, and multiple sclerosis.
- Rare Diseases: Finding new uses for drugs to treat rare or orphan diseases, which may lack dedicated treatments.
- Mental Health Conditions: Repurposing drugs to manage mental health disorders such as depression, anxiety, and PTSD.

CHALLENGES AND CONSIDERATIONS

As drug repurposing advances, there are challenges and considerations to address:

- Regulatory Approval: Navigating regulatory pathways for repurposed drugs, which may require different data and evidence than new drugs.

- Intellectual Property: Managing intellectual property rights and patents when repurposing drugs.

- Clinical Trial Design: Designing clinical trials to test repurposed drugs effectively and efficiently.

- Safety and Efficacy: Ensuring the safety and efficacy of repurposed drugs for new indications.

- Cost and Accessibility: Balancing the cost and accessibility of repurposed drugs, especially in low-income regions.

LAB-ON-A-CHIP: REVOLUTIONIZING DIAGNOSTICS AND RESEARCH

Lab-on-a-chip (LOC) technology integrates multiple laboratory processes onto a single chip, enabling precise and efficient analysis in a compact and portable format. This groundbreaking technology is transforming diagnostics, research, and personalized medicine by enabling rapid and accurate testing with minimal sample and reagent usage. In this chapter, we will explore the future of lab-on-a-chip technology, highlighting emerging trends and concrete examples of how it is revolutionizing diagnostics and research.

UNDERSTANDING LAB-ON-A-CHIP TECHNOLOGY

Lab-on-a-chip technology miniaturizes laboratory processes onto a small chip:

- Microfluidics: The manipulation of small volumes of fluids in micro-scale channels for precise control and analysis.

- Multi-Functionality: Integrating multiple laboratory functions, such as sample preparation, separation, and detection, onto a single chip.

- Portable Diagnostics: Enabling point-of-care testing with compact devices that can be used outside traditional lab settings.

- Automated Analysis: Performing complex assays and analysis automatically on the chip, reducing the need for manual intervention.

- High Throughput: Processing multiple samples or conducting multiple assays simultaneously for increased efficiency.

EMERGING TRENDS IN LAB-ON-A-CHIP TECHNOLOGY

Several trends are shaping the future of lab-on-a-chip technology:

- AI and Machine Learning Integration: Utilizing AI and machine learning to analyze data from LOC devices and provide actionable insights.

- Wearable LOC Devices: Developing wearable devices with integrated LOC technology for continuous health monitoring.

- 3D Printing and Fabrication: Utilizing 3D printing for rapid prototyping and manufacturing of LOC devices.

- Miniaturized Sensing Technologies: Incorporating advanced sensors such as biosensors and optical sensors for enhanced detection capabilities.

- Multiplexed Assays: Designing LOC systems that can conduct multiple tests simultaneously for comprehensive analysis.

APPLICATIONS OF LAB-ON-A-CHIP TECHNOLOGY

Lab-on-a-chip technology is transforming various aspects of diagnostics and research:

- Point-of-Care Testing: Providing rapid and accurate diagnostics at the point of care, including for infectious diseases and chronic conditions.

- Genetic Testing: Enabling genetic analysis and screening with minimal sample sizes and quick turnaround times.

- Drug Development: Facilitating high-throughput screening and testing of drug candidates on a single chip.

- Environmental Monitoring: Detecting pollutants, toxins, and other environmental hazards with portable LOC devices.

- Personalized Medicine: Supporting personalized treatment plans with rapid diagnostic testing and biomarker analysis.

CHALLENGES AND CONSIDERATIONS

As lab-on-a-chip technology advances, there are challenges and considerations to address:

- Integration with Healthcare Systems: Ensuring LOC devices can integrate seamlessly with electronic health records and other healthcare technologies.

- Manufacturing and Cost: Developing cost-effective manufacturing processes to make LOC devices accessible to a wide range of users.

- Regulation and Standardization: Establishing clear guidelines and standards for LOC devices to ensure safety and reliability.

- Data Security and Privacy: Protecting patient data and ensuring secure communication within LOC systems.

- Scalability and Customization: Balancing scalability with the need for customized LOC devices for specific applications.

WEARABLE HEALTH TECH: THE FUTURE OF PERSONAL HEALTH MONITORING

Wearable health technology is revolutionizing healthcare by providing individuals with real-time monitoring and insights into their health and well-being. These devices, which include smartwatches, fitness trackers, and other wearable sensors, offer a convenient and personalized way to track vital signs, activity levels, sleep patterns, and more. In this chapter, we will explore the future of wearable health tech, highlighting emerging trends and concrete examples of how these innovations are reshaping the healthcare landscape.

EVOLUTION OF WEARABLE HEALTH TECH

Wearable health tech has evolved from simple pedometers to sophisticated devices that can monitor a wide range of health metrics. Key milestones in the evolution of wearable health tech include:

- Activity Trackers: Early wearables focused on tracking physical activity, such as step count, distance, and calories burned.

- Heart Rate Monitors: Wearables began incorporating heart rate sensors to monitor cardiovascular health during exercise and throughout the day.

- Sleep Trackers: Advanced wearables can track sleep duration and quality, providing insights into sleep patterns and potential disruptions.

- ECG and Blood Pressure Monitors: Some wearables now offer medical-grade sensors for monitoring electrocardiograms (ECGs) and blood pressure.

INNOVATIVE APPLICATIONS OF WEARABLE HEALTH TECH

Wearable health tech is expanding beyond basic monitoring to offer more advanced and personalized applications:

- Stress and Emotion Tracking: Wearables equipped with sensors can detect changes in skin conductance and heart rate variability, providing insights into stress levels and emotional states.

- Respiratory Health Monitoring: Wearables with respiratory sensors can monitor breathing patterns and detect potential issues such as sleep apnea.

- Glucose Monitoring: Non-invasive glucose monitoring is an emerging area of wearable tech that could benefit individuals with diabetes.

- Wearable Patches: Adhesive patches with sensors can continuously monitor specific health metrics, such as hydration levels and body temperature.

INTEGRATION WITH HEALTHCARE SYSTEMS

Wearable health tech is increasingly being integrated with healthcare systems to improve patient care and outcomes:

- Remote Patient Monitoring: Wearables allow healthcare providers to remotely monitor patients' health metrics, enabling early intervention and personalized treatment adjustments.
- AI-Driven Insights: Wearable data can be analyzed using artificial intelligence (AI) algorithms to identify trends, predict health risks, and offer personalized health recommendations.
- Telehealth and Wearable Tech: Combining telehealth consultations with wearable data provides a comprehensive view of a patient's health and supports more informed decision-making.

FUTURE TRENDS IN WEARABLE HEALTH TECH

The future of wearable health tech holds exciting possibilities:

- Wearable Implants: Wearable implants, such as biosensors, could provide continuous monitoring of internal health metrics and offer targeted therapies.

- Smart Clothing: Integration of sensors into clothing could enable seamless monitoring of multiple health metrics without the need for additional devices.

- Wearable Brain-Computer Interfaces: Wearables may extend to brain-computer interfaces, allowing for real-time monitoring and potential therapeutic applications for neurological conditions.

- Advanced AI and Wearables: AI will continue to play a key role in analyzing wearable data, offering more precise health insights and recommendations.

CHALLENGES AND CONSIDERATIONS

While wearable health tech offers many benefits, there are challenges and considerations to address:

- Data Privacy and Security: Protecting the privacy of wearable data is essential, as it can reveal sensitive information about an individual's health.

- Accuracy and Reliability: Ensuring the accuracy and reliability of wearable sensors is crucial for meaningful health insights.

- Regulation and Approval: Regulatory bodies must establish clear guidelines for the safety and efficacy of wearable health tech.

- Accessibility and Affordability: Making wearable health tech accessible and affordable to all individuals is important for equitable healthcare.

GLOSSARY

A

- AI (Artificial Intelligence): The use of computer algorithms and models to simulate human intelligence and automate decision-making processes.

- Augmented Reality (AR): An interactive experience where digital information is overlaid on the real-world environment.

B

- Biocompatibility: The ability of a material or device to be safely used in the body without causing adverse reactions.

- Bioprinting: The process of creating three-dimensional tissues or organs using bioinks and specialized printers.

- Biosensors: Devices that detect biological molecules or processes and provide a measurable signal.

C

- Controlled Release: A method of delivering drugs in a controlled manner over time.

- Crowdsourcing: The practice of obtaining input, ideas, or solutions from a large group of people, often through the internet.

D

- Drug Repurposing (Repositioning): The process of finding new uses for existing medications beyond their original indications.

G

- Gamification: The use of game design elements to make activities more engaging and motivating.

- Genomics: The study of an organism's complete set of DNA, including genes and their functions.

H

- High-Throughput Screening: A process of rapidly testing a large number of compounds or samples for a specific biological activity.

I

- Immunotherapy: A type of treatment that uses the body's immune system to fight diseases, particularly cancer.

L

- Lab-on-a-Chip (LOC): Technology that integrates multiple laboratory processes onto a single chip for rapid and efficient analysis.

M

- Machine Learning: A subset of AI that involves training algorithms to learn patterns from data and make predictions or decisions.
- Microbiome: The community of microorganisms, such as bacteria, fungi, and viruses, that live on or within the human body.

- Microfluidics: The manipulation of small volumes of fluids in micro-scale channels for precise control and analysis.

- Multiplexed Assays: Assays that allow for the simultaneous testing of multiple targets or conditions.

N

- Nanoparticles: Tiny particles, often between 1 and 100 nanometers in size, that can carry drugs or other substances for targeted delivery.

- Nanoscale Drug Delivery: The use of nanoparticles to deliver drugs precisely to targeted cells and tissues in the body.

- Nanotechnology: The manipulation and use of materials at the nanoscale for various applications.

- Nutrigenomics: The study of how genes and nutrients interact to influence health and disease.

P

- Personalized Medicine: Tailoring medical treatments to an individual's genetic, molecular, and health profile.

- Precision Oncology: The use of personalized medicine in cancer treatment, targeting specific genetic mutations and biomarkers.

S

- Smart Pill Bottles: Medication containers equipped with technology to track and remind patients about their medication schedules.

T

- Therapeutic Gaming: The use of video games and gamified apps as therapeutic tools for mental health and rehabilitation.

- Virtual Reality (VR): An immersive, simulated experience that can replicate or transform real-world environments.

APPENDIX

A. ADDITIONAL RESOURCES

1. Books and Journals:

- Nature Biotechnology: A journal covering biotechnology and related fields, including research and innovation.

- Microbiome: A journal dedicated to the study of the human microbiome and its impact on health.

- The Personalized Medicine Revolution by Pieter Cullis: A book on the future of personalized medicine and how it will transform healthcare.

- The Patient Will See You Now by Eric Topol: A book on the future of medicine and the impact of technology on healthcare.

2. Online Courses and Tutorials:

- Coursera: Offers a wide range of courses on topics such as bioinformatics, genomics, and personalized medicine.

- edX: Provides courses on health technology, mental health, and drug development.

- FutureLearn: Offers courses on microbiome science and other emerging topics in healthcare.

3. Websites and Online Communities:

- National Institutes of Health (NIH): A comprehensive resource for information on medical research, clinical trials, and health news.

- World Health Organization (WHO): Provides updates on global health trends and emerging health technologies.

- American Association for the Advancement of Science (AAAS): Offers resources on recent scientific advancements.

B. FURTHER READING

1. Research Papers:

- Applications of Wearable Technology in Healthcare: A research paper discussing the latest advancements in wearable health tech.

- The Impact of Nanotechnology on Drug Delivery: An article exploring the potential of nanoscale drug delivery systems.

- Immunotherapy in Cancer Treatment: A review of the recent developments and future directions in cancer immunotherapy.

2. White Papers and Reports:

- Future of Healthcare Technology: A report detailing trends and projections in medical technology.

- Precision Medicine and Genomics: A white paper discussing the integration of precision medicine and genomics in healthcare.

C. SUPPLEMENTARY INFORMATION

1. Glossary of Terms: Refer to the glossary section for a comprehensive list of key terms related to the topics covered in the book.

2. Abbreviations and Acronyms:

- AI: Artificial Intelligence

- AR: Augmented Reality

- LOC: Lab-on-a-Chip

- VR: Virtual Reality

3. Index:

- For ease of reference, use the index at the end of the book to locate specific topics and terms covered in the chapters.

4. Additional Notes:

- Ethics and Privacy: Considerations regarding the ethical use of emerging medical technologies and data privacy.

- Patient Education: Resources for educating patients about new medical treatments and health technologies.

DISCLAIMER

The information presented in this book is intended for general educational and informational purposes only. It is not intended as medical advice, diagnosis, or treatment. Always seek the advice of your physician or another qualified healthcare provider regarding any medical condition or treatment options.

The content in this book is based on current research, scientific knowledge, and trends at the time of writing. AI technology was used in the research and generation of some content within this book. As medical science and technology are constantly evolving, some information may become outdated over time. Readers are advised to consult reliable sources and medical professionals for the most up-to-date information.

The author and publisher do not assume any liability for actions taken based on the information provided in this book. Use of the information contained in this book is at the reader's own risk. The author and publisher make no warranties, express or implied, regarding the accuracy, completeness, or reliability of the information provided.

Mention of any specific products, treatments, technologies, or services does not imply endorsement by the author or publisher. Readers are encouraged to conduct their own research and exercise critical thinking when making healthcare decisions.

This book may include discussions of scientific and medical research, including ongoing studies and experimental treatments. These discussions are for informational purposes only and do not imply the effectiveness or safety of any treatment or technology. Consult with a qualified healthcare provider for personalized medical advice and treatment options.

By reading this book, you acknowledge and agree to the terms of this disclaimer. Thank you for your understanding and for using the information in this book responsibly. Here's an updated disclaimer for your nonfiction book that includes the use of AI:

Disclaimer

The information presented in this book is intended for general educational and informational purposes only. It is not intended as medical advice, diagnosis, or treatment. Always seek the advice of your physician or another qualified healthcare provider regarding any medical condition or treatment options.

The content in this book is based on current research, scientific knowledge, and trends at the time of writing. AI technology was used in the research and generation of some content within this book. As medical science and technology are constantly evolving, some information may become outdated over time. Readers are advised to consult reliable sources and medical professionals for the most up-to-date information.

The author and publisher do not assume any liability for actions taken based on the information provided in this book. Use of the information contained in this book is at the reader's own risk. The author and publisher make no warranties, express or implied, regarding the accuracy, completeness, or reliability of the information provided.

Mention of any specific products, treatments, technologies, or services does not imply endorsement by the author or publisher. Readers are encouraged to conduct their own research and exercise critical thinking when making healthcare decisions.

This book may include discussions of scientific and medical research, including ongoing studies and experimental treatments. These discussions are for informational purposes only and do not imply the effectiveness or safety of any treatment or technology. Consult with a qualified healthcare provider for personalized medical advice and treatment options.

By reading this book, you acknowledge and agree to the terms of this disclaimer. Thank you for your understanding and for using the information in this book responsibly.

www.ingramcontent.com/pod-product-compliance
Lightning Source LLC
Chambersburg PA
CBHW070343230526
45471CB00006B/2424